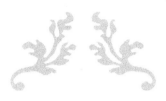

UNDERSTANDING
DIABETIC AIR FRYER

A Comprehensive Guide To The Best Diabetic Diet Recipes And
Balanced Meals To Set A Correct Diet And Regain a Healthy
Bodyweight

TASTY FOOD ACADEMY

This document is geared towards providing exact and reliable information in regard to the topic and issue covered.

- From a Declaration of Principles which was accepted and approved equally by a Committee of the American Bar Association and a Committee of Publishers and Associations.

Table of Contents

Introduction 8

Quick and Easy Recipes 11

    1. Apple Chips 12

    2. Veggie Quesadillas 14

    3. Greek Feta Fries 16

    4. Crispy Pork Belly Crack 18

    5. Crispy Garlic Keto Croutons 20

Breakfast Recipes 23

    6. Tomatoes and Cheese Frittata 24

    7. Egg White and Flax Crepes 26

    8. Scrambled Tofu 28

    9. Bell Pepper, Salsa, and Taco Frittata 30

    10. Breaded Squash Blooms 32

Snacks and Appetizer Recipes 34

    11. Air Fryer Soft Pretzels 35

    12. Air Fryer Blackberry Hand Pies 38

    13. Air Fryer Biscuits 41

    14. Air Fryer Churros with Chocolate Sauce 43

    15. Air Fryer Strawberry Pop-Tarts 45

Pork, Beef and Lamb Recipes 48

    16. Cheesy Beef Paseíllo 49

    17. Pork Head Chops with Vegetables 51

    18. Flavored Pork Chops 53

    19. Meatloaf Reboot 54

    20. Mediterranean Lamb Meatballs 55

Fish & Seafood Recipes 58

21. Garlic Rosemary Grilled Prawns.. 59

22. Air-Fried Crumbed Fish 61

23. Parmesan Garlic Crusted Salmon... 62

24. Air Fryer Salmon with Maple Soy Glaze..................................... 64

Poultry Recipes 67

25. Chicken Meatballs.. 68

26. Buffalo Chicken Hot Wings 70

27. Chicken with Cashew Nuts.. 72

28. Fried Chicken Tamari and Mustard... 74

29. Herbed Chicken.. 76

30. Chinese Stuffed Chicken 78

Vegetables and Sides Recipes.. 81

31. Kiwi Chips... 82

32. Apple Crisp... 83

33. Roasted Veggies... 85

34. Sweet and Spicy Carrots 87

35. Air Fried Potatoes 89

36. Asparagus Avocado Soup... 90

Dessert Recipes... 93

37. Sugar-Free Low Carb Peanut Butter Cookies............................. 94

38. Air Fryer Blueberry Muffins 96

39. Air Fryer Sugar-Free Lemon Slice and Bake Cookies................... 98

40. Easy Air Fryer Brownies 100

Conclusion 103

Introduction

As a diabetic, you face unique challenges while cooking. For example, you need to be careful about what you eat, but it's also important to eat healthily. You can cook healthy food with a device that helps manage your diabetes. Air fryers are one such device you can use to air fry foods without deep-frying or using oil or any other unhealthy methods.

An air fryer is a cooking device that uses a reduced quantity of oil and dry air in a high temperature to cook food. Using an air fryer is fast as you don't need to cook your food for a long time; it heats up the air quickly while the food cooks. You don't need to pre-heat or make any preparation before using this device.

If you like to enjoy fried food but don't want to suffer the effect of eating trans-fat and artificial oils, then you should try cooking with an air fryer.

Fat is an essential component that plays a vital role in a healthy diet. Fats provide essential fatty acids and energy that are both important for the body. They help regulate cholesterol metabolism and maintain healthy skin. Dietary fats facilitate the absorption of fat-soluble vitamins and hormones to satisfy people's appetite.

You will also learn how to make real-life recipes with air fryers that help you manage your diabetes and improve your health at the same time. You will learn how to prepare delicious recipes that work with any type of food, dish, or meal you want to prepare at home or at your favorite restaurant.

You don't have to spend hours in the kitchen preparing delicious meals. With its rapid cooking time of five to twenty minutes, you can have freshly cooked food with little effort.

Quick and Easy Recipes

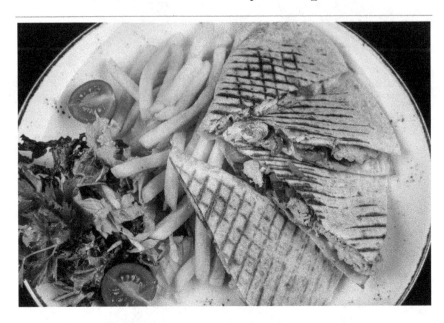

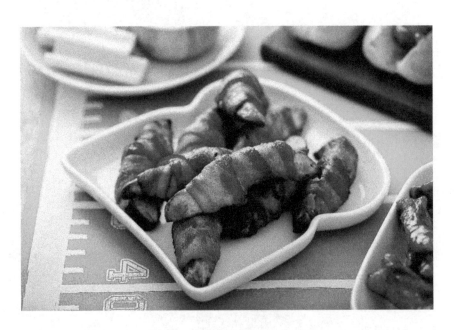

1. Apple Chips

Preparation Time: 6 minutes

Cooking Time: 18 minutes

Servings: 4

Ingredients:

- Cooking spray
- 2 tsp. canola oil
- ¼ cup plain low-fat Greek yogurt
- 1 tsp. honey
- 1 tsp. ground cinnamon
- 1 tbsp. almond butter
- 1 apple

Directions:

1. Slice the apple into thin slices.
2. Mix the slices of apple with oil and cinnamon before you toss them together for even coating.
3. Apply cooking spray on your air fryer basket.
4. Place the slices of apple in the air fryer basket. Don't place more than 8 slices on a single layer.
5. Cook the apple at 375°F for 12 minutes. Ensure you rearrange the slices of apple after every 4 minutes. It is possible that the apple chips are not crispy enough when you remove them

from your air fryer. They will become even crispier as they cool.

6. If there are slices of apple left, you can do the same thing to them.

7. Mix the honey, almond butter, and yogurt together evenly. Add a dollop of the sauce to every serving of the apple chips.

Nutrition:

- **Calories**: 104 kcal
- **Fat**: 3 g
- **Carbohydrates**: 2 g
- **Proteins**: 1 g

2. Veggie Quesadillas

Preparation Time: 21 minutes

Cooking Time: 18 minutes

Servings: 4

Ingredients:

- Cooking spray
- 4 sprouted whole-grain flour tortillas
- 4 ounces reduced-fat sharp Cheddar cheese, shredded (about 1 cup)
- 2 tbsp. chopped fresh cilantro
- 2 ounces plain reduced-fat Greek yogurt
- ¼ tsp. ground cumin
- ½ cup drained refrigerated Pico de gallo
- 1 tsp. lime zest plus 1 tbsp. fresh juice (from 1 lime)
- 1 cup sliced zucchini
- 1 cup sliced red bell pepper
- 1 cup no-salt-added canned black beans, drained, and rinsed

Directions:

1. Sprinkle 2 tbsp. of shredded cheese over half of each tortilla. After that, you can add cheese on the tortilla. Also, add black beans, slices of zucchini, and a quarter cup of red pepper slices on the tortilla as well.

2. Sprinkle the remaining cheese on the tortilla. Now, you can fold the tortilla in the shape of half-moon. They will now become quesadillas. We hope you understand that quesadillas are tortillas with fillings.

3. Coat the quesadillas with cooking spray and secure them with toothpicks.

4. Coat the air fryer basket with cooking spray. Then, you can place the quesadillas in the basket. Cook them at 400°F until they turn golden brown and crispy. This should happen after about 10 minutes of cooking. Remember to turn the quesadillas over after 5 minutes. You can air fry all the quesadillas at once or in two batches.

5. While the quesadillas are being cooked, mix the cumin, lime juice, lime zest, and yogurt together in a bowl.

6. You need to cut each of the quesadillas into wedges before you serve them. It is also necessary to sprinkle cilantro on them. Serve each of them with a tbsp. of cumin and 2 tbsp. of Pico de Gallo

Nutrition:

- **Calories**: 291 kcal
- **Fat**: 8 g
- **Carbohydrates**: 12 g
- **Proteins**: 17 g

3. Greek Feta Fries

Preparation Time: 12 minutes

Cooking Time: 15-20 minutes

Servings: 2

Ingredients:

- Cooking spray
- 2potatoes, scrubbed and dried
- 1 tbsp. olive oil
- 2 tsp. lemon zest
- ½ tsp. dried oregano
- ¼ tsp. kosher salt
- ¼ tsp. garlic powder
- ¼ tsp. onion powder
- ¼ tsp. paprika
- ¼ tsp. black pepper
- 2 ounces feta cheese, finely grated (about ½ cup)
- 2 ounces shredded skinless rotisserie chicken breast
- ¼ cup prepared tzatziki
- ¼ cup seeded and diced plum tomato
- 2 tbsp. chopped red onion
- 1 tbsp. chopped fresh flat-leaf parsley and oregano

Directions:

1. Preheat an air fryer to 380°F. Coat the basket with cooking spray. Now, you should cut each potato into ¼-inch thick slices.

2. Mix the potatoes together with some oil. Add the pepper, paprika, onion powder, garlic powder, salt, and dried oregano together with zest. Season the potatoes with the zest mixture.

3. Air fry the potatoes for about 7 minutes. Turn them over and cook them for another 8 minutes. The potatoes should be crispy by then.

4. Remove the potato fries and top it with herbs, red onion, tomato, remaining feta, chicken, and tzatziki. You can now serve the meal.

Nutrition:

- **Calories**: 383 kcal
- **Fat**: 16 g
- **Carbohydrates**: 20 g
- **Proteins**: 19 g

4. Crispy Pork Belly Crack

Preparation Time: 5 minutes

Cooking Time: 25 minutes

Servings: 4

Ingredients:

- ½ tsp. pepper
- 1 tsp. sea salt
- 1 lb. raw pork belly strips

Directions:

1. Start by slicing the pork belly strips. The idea is to cut the pork into sizes that can be chewed easily.
2. Mix the salt and pepper tighter evenly in a small bowl.
3. Put the pieces of pork belly in the mixture and toss them for even coating.
4. Preheat your air fryer for about 3 minutes
5. Now, put the pieces of pork in your air fryer basket.
6. Set the temperature to about 390°F and cook the pork for about 15 minutes, but make sure you turn them over every 5 minutes.
7. After 15 minutes, they should be crispy and done.
8. Sometimes, they may take a little longer, or they could take less than 15 minutes. That's why you need to keep checking them every 5 minutes.

9. Drain them on paper towels. Now, you can serve them either hot or warm. Enjoy your tasty meal. You can add more spices to yours. Cooking requires being creative.

Nutrition:

- **Calories**: 332 kcal
- **Fat**: 24 g
- **Carbohydrates**: 20 g
- **Proteins**: 26 g

5. Crispy Garlic Keto Croutons

Preparation Time: 12 minutes

Cooking Time: 10 minutes

Serving: 1

Ingredients:

- 2 tbsp. Olive Oil
- 2 Cups Keto Farmers Bread or half of the loaf
- ½ tbsp. garlic powder
- 1 tbsp. Marjoram

Directions:

1. Cut your bread into several slices and cut each slice into smaller squares.

2. Place the pieces of bread into a bowl and add the other three ingredients to it. Mix them together.

3. Now, pour the croutons mixture into your air fryer basket. Make sure everything is on a single layer for crispiness. Don't add additional oil. An air fryer works best with little oil.

4. Air fry the bread for about 10 minutes to make it crispy. However, you need to shake it after 5 minutes. We suggest you select medium to high heat.

5. After about 10 minutes, the croutons should be ready for consumption.

6. Remove the croutons and give them 5 minutes to cool down before you serve them.

7. Enjoy the recipe!

Nutrition:

- **Calories**: 50 kcal
- **Fat**: 4 g
- **Carbohydrates**: 1 g
- **Proteins**: 2 g

Breakfast Recipes

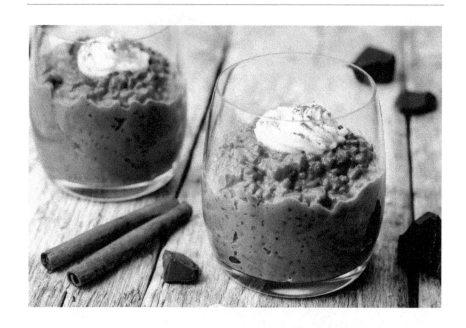

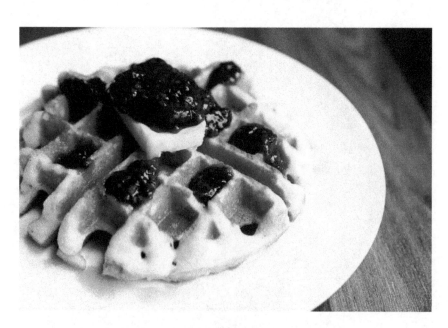

6. Tomatoes and Cheese Frittata

Preparation Time: 7 minutes

Cooking Time: 10 minutes

Servings: 4

Ingredients:

- 8 eggs
- 2 tomatoes
- ¼ cup milk, fat-free
- ½ cup cheddar cheese, reduced-fat
- 2 leeks, sliced
- 1 tbsp. fresh thyme
- Pinch salt
- Pinch pepper

Directions:

1. Preheat the Air Fryer to 330°F.
2. In a baking dish, grease leeks with olive oil. Add eggs, cheese, salt, and pepper. Layer tomato slices on top.
3. Place baking dish onside the Air fryer basket. Cook for 10 minutes.
4. Remove and transfer the frittata to a plate. Sprinkle with thyme. Serve.

Nutrition:

- **Calories**: 186
- **Fat**: 11.1 g
- **Carbohydrates**: 9.1 g
- **Proteins**: 11.9 g

7. Egg White and Flax Crepes

Preparation Time: 8 minutes

Cooking Time: 26 minutes

Servings: 3

Ingredients:

- 3 egg whites only
- 2 tbsp. ground flaxseed
- 2 eggs
- ¼ cup coconut flour
- ¼ cup almond milk
- ½ tsp. baking soda

Directions:

1. Combine all ingredients in a food processor or blender and blend until thoroughly combined.
2. Pour batter into the air fryer hot skillet covered with cooking spray and swirl around to create a large, thin circle.
3. Let cook until bubbles in the batter begin to pop, gently easing up the sides every few moments, about 3 minutes or less.
4. Flip crepes and cook on the other side until firm. Serve.

Nutrition:

- **Calories**: 78.7
- **Fat**: 5.3 g
- **Carbohydrates**: 5.5 g
- **Proteins**: 3.1 g

8. Scrambled Tofu

Preparation Time: 7 minutes

Cooking Time: 10-12 minutes

Servings: 2

Ingredients:

- 4-6 whole wheat tortillas, warmed
- 2 14-ounce blocks extra-firm tofu
- 1 15-ounce can black beans, rinsed, drained
- 2 tbsp. vegetable oil
- 1 onion, chopped
- ½ tsp. ground cumin
- ½ tsp. ground coriander
- 1 green bell pepper, chopped finely
- 1 red bell pepper, chopped finely
- 1 ½ tsp. ground turmeric
- ¼ cup coarsely chopped fresh cilantro
- Salt
- Ground pepper

Garnishes:

- Salsa
- scallions, sliced
- Cheddar, grated

- Avocado, chopped

Directions:

1. Place tofu on a plate lined with several layers of paper towels. Smash tofu using a fork or potato masher.
2. Put onion and peppers in the Air fryer basket. Cook for 2 minutes. Season with cumin and coriander. Cook for 1 minute.
3. Add in tofu. Stir in turmeric. Add beans; cook, often stirring, until heated through, 1–2 minutes. Stir in cilantro; season with salt and pepper.
4. Serve scrambled with tortillas and garnishes, as desired.

Nutrition:

- **Calories**: 100
- **Fat**: 5 g
- **Carbohydrates**: 6 g
- **Proteins**: 8 g

9. Bell Pepper, Salsa, and Taco Frittata

Preparation Time: 11 minutes

Cooking Time: 24 minutes

Servings: 4

Ingredients:

- 6 eggs
- ¾ cup cheddar cheese, reduced-fat
- ¼ cup onions, chopped
- ¼ cup green bell peppers, chopped
- 1 cup salsa
- 2 tbsp. taco seasoning
- 1 cup sour cream, low fat
- 1 oz. milk, low fat
- Pinch salt
- Pinch pepper

Directions:

1. Preheat USA Air Fryer to 330°F.
2. Combine eggs, green bell pepper, taco seasoning, onions, milk, cheddar cheese, salt, and pepper in a bowl.
3. Transfer mixture to a baking dish. Lightly grease with cooking spray. Put baking dish inside the Air Fryer basket. Cook for 20 minutes.
4. Top with salsa and sour cream. Serve.

Nutrition:

- **Calories**: 140
- **Fat**: 17 g
- **Carbohydrates**: 5.3 g
- **Proteins**: 17.6 g

10. Breaded Squash Blooms

Preparation Time: 10 minutes

Cooking Time: 24 minutes

Servings: 3

Ingredients:

- 2½ pounds squash flowers, rinsed
- 1 cup coconut flour, finely milled
- Pinch sea salt, to taste
- raisin vinegar for garnish, optional

Directions:

1. Preheat Air Fryer to 330°F.
2. Season squash blossoms with salt. Dredge into coconut flour.
3. Layer breaded blossoms in the air fryer basket. Fry for 2 minutes or until golden brown. Drain on paper towels.
4. Stack cooked squash blossoms in the middle of plates. Sprinkle raisin vinegar. Serve.

Nutrition:

- **Calories**: 5
- **Fat**: 0.2 g
- **Carbohydrates**: 1 g
- **Proteins**: 0.1 g

Snacks and Appetizer Recipes

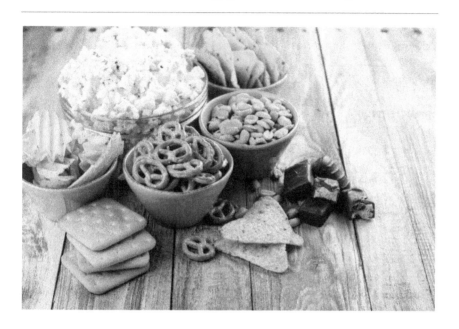

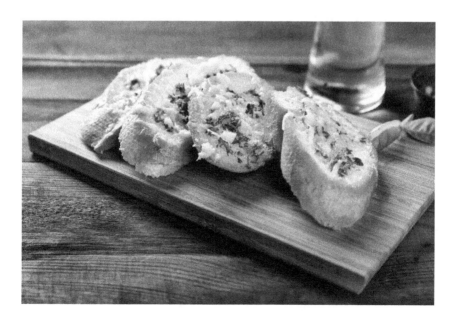

11. Air Fryer Soft Pretzels

Preparation Time: 9 minutes

Cooking Time: 18 minutes

Servings: 12

Ingredients:

- 1 ½ cups warm
- 2 tsp. kosher salt
- 1 tbsp. sugar
- 1 package active dry yeast
- 2 ounces melted butter
- 4 ½ cups all-purpose flour
- 2/3 cup baking soda
- 10 cups water
- 1 egg yolk
- Pretzel salt

Directions:

1. In a bowl of your stand mixer fitted with a dough hook, mix the water, salt, and sugar together. Sprinkle on top with yeast and let sit for five minutes.
2. Pour the flour into the bowl and add the butter; combine the mixture together at low speed.

3. Increase the speed to medium and knead the dough for 5 minutes until smooth and does not stick to the side of the bowl.
4. Transfer the dough to a greased bowl; cover with plastic wrap. Let dough sit for 50 to 60 minutes at a warm temperature until the size has doubled.
5. Prepare two baking sheets and line them with parchment paper and then mist with nonstick spray.
6. Heat up your air fryer at 400°F.
7. Meanwhile, combine in a large roasting pan or stockpot the baking soda and 10 cups of water; bring to a boil.
8. Lay the pretzel dough on a greased work surface and equally divide into 12 pieces. Roll each dough piece into an 18" rope and then twist to form into a pretzel shape.
9. Working on each piece of pretzel, place in the boiling water for thirty seconds and quickly remove from water. Transfer the pretzels to the prepared baking sheet.
10. Beat the egg yolk in 1 tbsp. of water and brush over the pretzels.
11. Sprinkle the pretzels with pretzel salt and load about 3 to 4 pieces into the air fryer basket. Cook for 6 minutes at 400°F; turn over and cook for additional 6 minutes or until dark golden brown.
12. Serve!

Nutrition:

- **Calories**: 214 kcal
- **Fat**: 4.7 g
- **Carbohydrates**: 17 g
- **Proteins**: 5.3 g

12. Air Fryer Blackberry Hand Pies

Preparation Time: 11 minutes

Cooking Time: 13 minutes

Servings: 6

Ingredients:

- 1 package refrigerated pie dough
- 1 beaten egg

For the filling:

- 12 ounces fresh blackberries
- 3 tbsp. all-purpose flour
- ¼ cup sugar
- ½ tsp. cinnamon
- 2 tbsp. lemon juice

For the icing:

- 1 cup powdered sugar
- ½ lemon

Directions:

1. Preheat your air fryer.
2. For the filling:

3. Wash the blackberries in running water. Transfer to a plate lined with a paper towel to drain excess water. Let it sit for one hour to dry completely.

4. Cut the fruits in half and transfer to a medium-sized bowl.

5. Add the sugar, flour, cinnamon, and lemon juice to the bowl with strawberries, tossing to combine well.

6. Pour the blackberry mixture into a medium-sized pot and cook on medium heat.

7. Using a potato masher, mash the berries until somewhat chunky. Turn off heat.

8. Set aside.

9. For the pie:

10. Dust the countertop with flour and lay the pie crusts on top. Roll the crusts out to ¼-inch thickness.

11. Cut out six circles from the crusts using a large circle cutter. Arrange the dough circles on a baking sheet.

12. Fill the dough with one tbsp. filling and brush the sides with beaten egg.

13. Fold the pie dough over, pressing down with your fingers to seal tightly. Leave indentations on the sides of the dough by pressing the edges with fork tines.

14. Using a pastry brush, lightly paint the top of the pies with beaten egg and lightly sprinkle with sugar.

15. Cook two pieces of pie dough at a time in the air fryer for 8 to 10 minutes at 380°F or until flaky and golden brown.

16. For the icing:

17. Put the sugar and lemon in a small bowl, whisking until combined. Slightly cool and top the hand pies with an icing drizzle.

18. Serve!

Nutrition:

- **Calories:**292 kcal
- **Fat**: 8 g
- **Carbohydrates**: 21 g
- **Proteins**: 3 g

13. Air Fryer Biscuits

Preparation Time: 12 minutes

Cooking Time: 13 minutes

Servings: 8

Ingredients:

- 175 grams self-rising flour
- 1 tsp. mustard powder
- 1 tbsp. thyme
- Pinch salt
- Dash pepper
- 25 grams butter
- 75 grams grated cheddar cheese
- 1 medium egg
- 30 ml whole milk

Directions:

1. Combine in a large mixing bowl the butter, flour, mustard powder, thyme, salt, and pepper.
2. With your hands, rub the fat into the flour mixture to form into coarse breadcrumbs.
3. Add in the whole milk, egg, and cheese to the flour mixture, mix with a fork and then finally mix it with your hands to form a large biscuit dough ball.
4. Dust your work surface with a little flour.

5. Roll out the dough ball with a rolling pin. Using biscuit cutters, form the dough into biscuit rounds.

6. Arrange the biscuit rounds in the air fryer grill pan at least 1 inch apart as they grow during cooking.

7. Cook the biscuits for 8 minutes at 360°F. Serve hot over the stew.

Nutrition:

- **Calories:**151 kcal
- **Fat:** 7 g
- **Carbohydrates:** 16 g
- **Proteins:** 6 g

14. Air Fryer Churros with Chocolate Sauce

Preparation Time: 6 minutes

Cooking Time: 27 minutes

Servings: 12

Ingredients:

- ½ cup water
- ¼ cup, plus 2 tbsp. unsalted butter, divided
- ¼ tsp. kosher salt
- 2 large eggs
- ½ cup all-purpose flour
- 2 tsp. ground cinnamon
- 1/3 cup granulated sugar
- 3 tbsp. heavy cream
- 4 ounces finely chopped bittersweet baking chocolate
- 2 tbsp. vanilla kefir

Directions:

1. In a small saucepan, bring ¼ cup of butter, salt, and water to a boil on medium-high heat.
2. Stir in flour vigorously using a wooden spoon form thirty seconds on medium-low heat.
3. Stir and cook for 2 to 3 minutes until the dough starts to detach from the sides of the saucepan and film formation is beginning to develop on the bottom of your pan.

4. Place the dough in a medium-size bowl, frequently stirring, for 1 minute until slightly cooled.

5. Add the eggs to the dough one at a time, often stirring, until the mixture is smooth.

6. Pour the mixture into a piping bag attached with a medium-sized star tip. Refrigerate for half an hour.

7. Pipe about six pieces with a length of 3 inches in an air fryer basket; make sure to arrange them in a single layer.

8. Cook the batter at 380°F for ten minutes until nicely golden. Do the rest of the remaining batter. In a medium bowl, mix the cinnamon and sugar.

9. Brush the cooked churros with 2 tbsp. of melted butter; roll churros in sugar mixture until well coated.

10. Put together in a small microwave-proof bowl the bittersweet baking chocolate and heavy cream. Microwave the mixture for 30 seconds on high until smooth and melted. Stir after fifteen seconds and add the kefir.

11. Serve with chocolate sauce.

Nutrition:

- **Calories**:173 kcal
- **Fat**: 11 g
- **Carbohydrates**: 12 g
- **Proteins**: 3 g

15. Air Fryer Strawberry Pop-Tarts

Preparation Time: 12 minutes

Cooking Time: 22 minutes

Servings: 6

Ingredients:

- ¼ cup granulated sugar
- 8 ounces quartered strawberries
- ½ (14.1 ounces) package refrigerated piecrusts
- Cooking spray
- 1 ½ tsp. fresh lemon juice from 1 lemon
- ½ cup powdered sugar
- ½ ounce rainbow candy sprinkles

Directions:

1. In a medium-size heatproof bowl, stir granulated sugar and strawberries until well coated. Let strawberry stand for 15 minutes, stirring often.

2. Microwave the sugarcoated strawberries on high for ten minutes until glossy and shrunk. Stir mixture halfway throughout cooking, let cool for half an hour.

3. Prepare the pie crust and roll into a twelve-inch circle on a surface lightly dusted with flour.

4. Cut the dough into 12 rectangular pieces, about 2 ½"by3" and reroll the scraps.

5. Fill the center of six of the rectangular pieces with two tsp. of strawberry mixture. Leave at least half-inch allowance on the border.

6. Brush the edges of dough rectangles with water and cover the filling with another piece of the dough rectangle. Press the edges of the dough with fork tines to seal completely. Coat the tarts with cooking spray.

7. Place three pieces of tarts in a single layer of your air fryer basket. Cook for ten minutes at 350°F until golden brown.

8. Repeat the same steps for the rest of the tart. Let cool on a wire rack for half an hour.

9. Prepare the glaze by stirring the sugar in lemon juice until smooth and spoon into cooled tarts.

10. Evenly sprinkle on top with candy sprinkles.

11. Serve!

Nutrition:

- **Calories**: 229 kcal
- **Fat**: 9 g
- **Carbohydrates**: 39 g
- **Proteins**: 2 g

Pork, Beef and Lamb Recipes

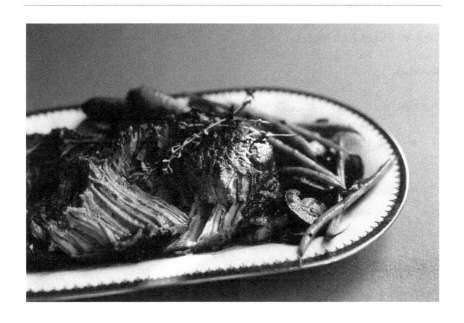

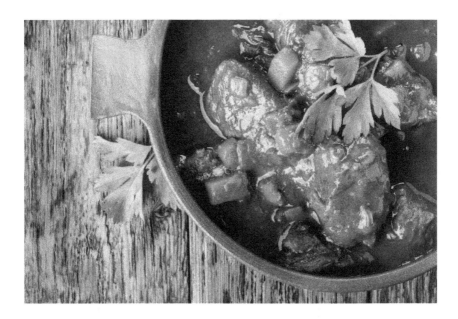

16. Cheesy Beef Paseíllo

Preparation Time: 9 minutes

Cooking Time: 23 minutes

Servings: 15

Ingredients:

- 1-2 tbsp. olive oil
- 2 pounds lean ground beef
- ½ chopped onion
- 2 cloves garlic, minced
- ½ tbsp. Adobo seasoning
- 2 tsp. dried oregano
- 1 packet optional seasoning
- 2 tbsp. chopped cilantro
- ¼ cup grated cheese
- 15 dough disks
- 15 slices yellow cheese

Directions:

1. In a large skillet over medium-high heat, heat the oil. Once the oil has warmed, add the meat, onions, and Adobo seasoning.

2. Brown veal, about 6–7 minutes. Drain the ground beef. Add the remaining seasonings and cilantro. Cook an additional minute. Add grated cheese, if desired. Melt the cheese.

3. On each dough disk, add a slice of cheese to the center and add 3-4 tbsp. of the meat mixture over the slice of cheese. Fold over the dough disk and with a fork, fold the edges and set it aside.

4. Preheat the air fryer to 370°F for 3 minutes.

5. Once three minutes have passed, spray the air fryer pan with cooking spray and add 3–4 cupcakes to the basket. Close the basket, set it to 370°F, and cook for 7 minutes. After 7 minutes, verify it. Cook up to 3 additional minutes, or the desired level of sharpness, if desired.

6. Repeat until finished.

Nutrition:

- **Calories**: 225 kcal
- **Fat**: 3.41 g
- **Carbohydrates**: 0 g
- **Proteins**: 20.9 g

17. Pork Head Chops with Vegetables

Preparation Time: 9 minutes

Cooking Time: 24 minutes

Servings: 4

Ingredients:

- 4 pork head chops
- 2 red tomatoes
- 1 large green pepper
- 4 mushrooms
- 1 onion
- 4 slices of cheese
- Salt
- Ground pepper
- Extra virgin olive oil

Directions:

1. Put the four chops on a plate and salt and pepper.
2. Put two of the chops in the air fryer basket.
3. Place tomato slices, cheese slices, pepper slices, onion slices and mushroom slices. Add some threads of oil.
4. Take the air fryer and select 180°C, 20 minutes.
5. Check that the meat is well made and take out.
6. Repeat the same operation with the other two pork chops.

Nutrition:

- **Calories**: 106 kcal
- **Fat**: 3.41 g
- **Carbohydrates**: 0 g
- **Proteins**: 20.9 g

18. Flavored Pork Chops

Preparation Time: 9 minutes

Cooking Time: 38 minutes

Servings: 2

Ingredients:

- 3 cloves ground garlic
- 2 tbsp. olive oil
- 1 tbsp. marinade
- 4 thawed pork chops

Directions:

1. Mix the cloves of ground garlic, marinade, and oil. Then apply this mixture on the chops.
2. Put the chops in the air fryer at 360°F for 35 minutes.

Nutrition:

- **Calories**: 118 kcal
- **Fat**: 3.41 g
- **Carbohydrates**: 0 g
- **Proteins**: 22 g

19. Meatloaf Reboot

Preparation Time: 13 minutes

Cooking Time: 10-15 minutes

Servings: 2

Ingredients:

- 4 slices leftover meatloaf, cut about 1-inch thick.

Directions:

1. Preheat your air fryer to 350°F.
2. Spray each side of the meatloaf slices with cooking spray. Add the slices to the air fryer and cook for about 9 to 10 minutes.
3. Don't turn the slices halfway through the cooking cycle because they may break apart. Instead, keep them on one side to cook to ensure they stay together

Nutrition:

- **Calories**: 201 kcal
- **Fat**: 5 g
- **Carbohydrates**: 9.6 g
- **Proteins**: 38 g

20. Mediterranean Lamb Meatballs

Preparation Time: 5 minutes

Cooking Time: 42 minutes

Servings: 4

Ingredients:

- 454 g ground lamb
- 3 cloves garlic, minced
- 5 g salt
- 1 g black pepper
- 2 g mint, freshly chopped
- 2 g ground cumin
- 3 ml hot sauce
- 1 g chili powder
- 1 scallion, chopped
- 8 g parsley, finely chopped
- 15 ml fresh lemon juice
- 2 g lemon zest
- 10 ml olive oil

Directions:

1. Mix the lamb, garlic, salt, pepper, mint, cumin, hot sauce, chili powder, chives, parsley, lemon juice, and lemon zest until well combined.

2. Create balls with the lamb mixture and cool for 30 minutes.

3. Select Preheat in the air fryer and press Start/Pause.

4. Cover the meatballs with olive oil and place them in the preheated fryer.

5. Select Steak, set the time to 10 minutes, and press Start/Pause.

Nutrition:

- **Calories**: 282 kcal
- **Fat**: 23.41 g
- **Carbohydrates**: 0.1 g
- **Proteins**: 16.59 g

Fish & Seafood Recipes

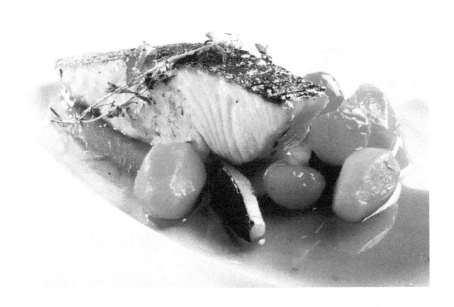

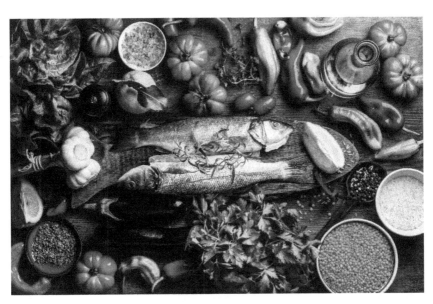

21. Garlic Rosemary Grilled Prawns

Preparation Time: 5 minutes

Cooking Time: 11 minutes

Servings: 2

Ingredients:

- Melted butter: ½ tbsp.
- Green capsicum: slices
- Eight prawns
- Rosemary leaves
- Kosher salt& freshly ground black pepper
- 3-4 cloves of minced garlic

Directions:

1. In a bowl, mix all the ingredients and marinate the prawns in it for at least 60 minutes or more
2. Add two prawns and two slices of capsicum on each skewer.
3. Let the air fryer preheat to 180 C.
4. Cook for 5-6 minutes. Then change the temperature to 200 C and cook for another minute.
5. Serve with lemon wedges.

Nutrition:

- **Calories**: 194 kcal
- **Fat**: 10 g
- **Carbohydrates**: 12 g
- **Proteins**: 26 g

22. Air-Fried Crumbed Fish

Preparation Time: 10 minutes

Cooking Time: 12 minutes

Servings: 2

Ingredients:

- Four fish fillets
- 4 tbsp. olive oil
- 1 egg beaten
- ¼ cup whole wheat breadcrumbs

Directions:

1. Let the air fryer preheat to 180 C.
2. In a bowl, mix breadcrumbs with oil. Mix well
3. First, coat the fish in the egg mix (egg mix with water), then in the breadcrumb mix. Coat well
4. Place in the air fryer, let it cook for 10-12 minutes.
5. Serve hot with salad green and lemon.

Nutrition:

- **Calories**: 254 kcal
- **Fat**: 12.7 g
- **Carbohydrates**: 10.2 g
- **Proteins**: 15.5 g

23. Parmesan Garlic Crusted Salmon

Preparation Time: 5 minutes

Cooking Time: 18 minutes

Servings: 2

Ingredients:

- Whole wheat breadcrumbs: ¼ cup
- 4 cups salmon
- 2 tbsp. butter, melted
- ¼ tsp. freshly ground black pepper
- ¼ cup Parmesan cheese (grated)
- 2 tsp. minced garlic
- ½ tsp. Italian seasoning

Directions:

1. Pat dry the salmon. In a bowl, mix Parmesan cheese, Italian seasoning, and breadcrumbs. In another pan, mix melted butter with garlic and add to the breadcrumbs mix. Mix well

2. Add kosher salt and freshly ground black pepper to salmon. On top of every salmon piece, add the crust mix and press gently.

3. Preheat let the air fryer to 400°F, spray the oil over the air fryer basket.

4. Cook salmon until done to your liking.

5. Serve hot with vegetable side dishes.

Nutrition:

- **Calories**: 330 kcal
- **Fat**: 19 g
- **Carbohydrates**: 11 g
- **Proteins**: 31 g

24. Air Fryer Salmon with Maple Soy Glaze

Preparation Time: 5 minutes

Cooking Time: 8 minutes

Servings: 4

Ingredients:

- 3 tbsp. pure maple syrup
- 3 tbsp. gluten-free soy sauce
- 1 tbsp. sriracha hot sauce
- 1 garlic clove, minced
- 4 salmon fillets, skinless

Directions:

1. In a Ziplock bag, mix sriracha, maple syrup, garlic, and soy sauce with salmon.
2. Mix well and let it marinate for at least half an hour.
3. Let the air fryer preheat to 400°F with oil spray the basket
4. Take fish out from the marinade, pat dry.
5. Put the salmon in the air fryer, cook for 7 to 8 minutes or longer.
6. In the meantime, in a saucepan, add the marinade, let it simmer until reduced to half.
7. Add glaze over salmon and serve.

Nutrition:

- **Calories**: 292 kcal
- **Fat**: 11 g
- **Carbohydrates**: 12 g
- **Proteins**: 35 g

Poultry Recipes

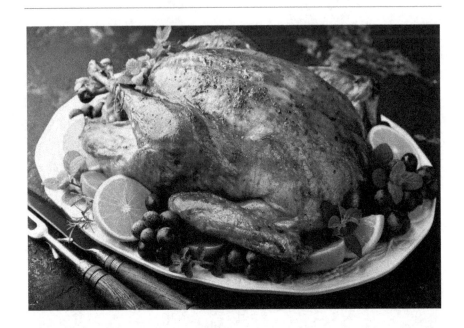

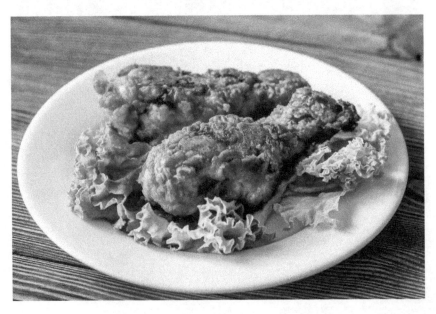

25. Chicken Meatballs

Preparation Time: 5 minutes

Cooking Time: 26 minutes

Servings: 4

Ingredients:

- 1-pound ground chicken
- 2 green onions, chopped
- ¾ tsp. ground black pepper
- ¼ cup shredded coconut, unsweetened
- 1 tsp. salt
- 1 tbsp. hoisin sauce
- 1 tbsp. soy sauce
- ½ cup cilantro, chopped
- 1 tsp. Sriracha sauce
- 1 tsp. sesame oil

Directions:

1. Switch on the air fryer, insert fryer basket, grease it with olive oil, then shut with its lid, set the fryer at 350°F and preheat for 5 minutes.
2. Meanwhile, place all the ingredients in a bowl, stir until well mixed and then shape the mixture into meatballs, 1 tsp. of chicken mixture per meatball.

3. Open the fryer, add chicken meatballs in a single layer, close with its lid and then spray with oil.

4. Cook the chicken meatballs for 10 minutes, flipping the meatballs halfway through, and then continue cooking for 3 minutes until golden.

5. When the air fryer beeps, open its lid, transfer chicken meatballs onto a serving plate and then cook the remaining meatballs in the same manner.

6. Serve straight away.

Nutrition:

- **Calories**: 223 kcal
- **Carbohydrates**: 3 g
- **Proteins**: 20 g
- **Fat**: 14 g

26. Buffalo Chicken Hot Wings

Preparation Time: 10 minutes

Cooking Time: 20-25 minutes

Servings: 6

Ingredients:

- 16 chicken wings, pastured
- 1 tsp. garlic powder
- 2 tsp. chicken seasoning
- ¾ tsp. ground black pepper
- 2 tsp. soy sauce
- ¼ cup buffalo sauce, reduced-fat

Directions:

1. Switch on the air fryer, insert fryer basket, grease it with olive oil, then shut with its lid, set the fryer at 400°F and preheat for 5 minutes.
2. Meanwhile, place chicken wings in a bowl, drizzle with soy sauce, toss until well coated, and then, season with black pepper and garlic powder.
3. Open the fryer, stack chicken wings in it, then spray with oil and close with its lid.
4. Cook the chicken wings for 10 minutes, turning the wings halfway through, and then transfer them to a bowl, covering the bowl with a foil to keep the chicken wings warm.

5. Air fry the remaining chicken wings in the same manner, then transfer them to the bowl, add buffalo sauce and toss until well coated.

6. Return chicken wings into the fryer basket in a single layer and continue frying for 7 to 12 minutes or until chicken wings are glazed and crispy, shaking the chicken wings every 3 to 4 minutes.

7. Serve straight away.

Nutrition:

- **Calories**: 88
- **Fat**: 6.5 g
- **Carbohydrates**: 2.6 g
- **Proteins**: 4.5 g

27. Chicken with Cashew Nuts

Preparation Time: 10 minutes

Cooking Time: 10-15 minutes

Servings: 4

Ingredients:

- 1 lb. chicken cubes
- 2 tbsp. soy sauce
- 1 tbsp. corn flour
- 2 ½ onion cubes
- 1 carrot, chopped
- 1/3 cup cashew nuts, fried
- 1 capsicum, cut
- 2 tbsp. garlic, crushed
- Salt and white pepper

Directions:

1. Marinate the chicken cubes with ½ tbsp. of white pepper, ½ tsp. salt, 2 tbsp. soya sauce, and add 1 tbsp. corn flour.

2. Set aside for 25 minutes. Preheat the Air Fryer to 380°F and transfer the marinated chicken. Add the garlic, the onion, the capsicum, and the carrot; fry for 5–6 minutes. Roll it in the cashew nuts before serving.

Nutrition:

- **Calories**: 425 kcal
- **Fat**: 35 g
- **Carbohydrates**: 25 g
- **Proteins**: 53 g

28. Fried Chicken Tamari and Mustard

Preparation Time: 10 minutes

Cooking Time: 30 minutes

Servings: 4

Ingredients:

- 1kg very small chopped chicken
- Tamari Sauce
- Original mustard
- Ground pepper
- 1 lemon
- Flour
- Extra virgin olive oil

Directions:

1. Put the chicken in a bowl; you can put the chicken with or without the skin to everyone's taste.
2. Add a generous stream of tamari, one or two tbsp. of mustard, a little ground pepper, and a splash of lemon juice.
3. Link everything very well and let macerate for an hour.
4. Pass the chicken pieces for flour and place them in the air fryer basket.
5. Put 20 minutes at 200°C. At halftime, move the chicken from the basket.

6. Do not crush the chicken; it is preferable to make two or three batches of chicken to pile up and do not fry the pieces well.

Nutrition:

- **Calories**: 100 kcal
- **Fat**: 6 g
- **Carbohydrates**: 0 g
- **Proteins**: 18 g

29. Herbed Chicken

Preparation Time: 10 minutes

Cooking Time: 40 minutes

Servings: 4

Ingredients:

- 1 whole chicken
- 1 tsp. garlic powder
- 1 tsp. onion powder
- ½ tsp. thyme; dried
- 1 tsp. rosemary; dried
- 1 tbsp. lemon juice
- 2 tbsp. olive oil
- Salt and black pepper to the taste

Directions:

1. Season chicken with salt and pepper, rub with thyme, rosemary, garlic powder, and onion powder, rub with lemon juice and olive oil and leave aside for 30 minutes.
2. Put the chicken in your air fryer and cook at 360°F for 20 minutes on each side. Leave chicken aside to cool down, carve and serve.

Nutrition:

- **Calories**: 390 kcal
- **Fat**: 10 g
- **Carbohydrates**: 22 g
- **Proteins**: 20 g

30. Chinese Stuffed Chicken

Preparation Time: 10 minutes

Cooking Time: 35-40 minutes

Servings: 8

Ingredients:

- 1 whole chicken
- 10 wolfberries
- 2 red chilies; chopped
- 4 ginger slices
- 1 yam; cubed
- 1 tsp. soy sauce
- 3 tsp. sesame oil
- Salt and white pepper to the taste

Directions:

1. Season chicken with salt, pepper, rub with soy sauce and sesame oil, and stuff with wolfberries, yam cubes, chilies, and ginger.
2. Place in your air fryer, cook at 400°F for 20 minutes, and then, at 360 F for 15 minutes. Carve chicken, divide among plates, and serve.

Nutrition:

- **Calories**: 320 kcal
- **Fat**: 12 g
- **Carbohydrates**: 22 g
- **Proteins**: 12 g

Vegetables and Sides Recipes

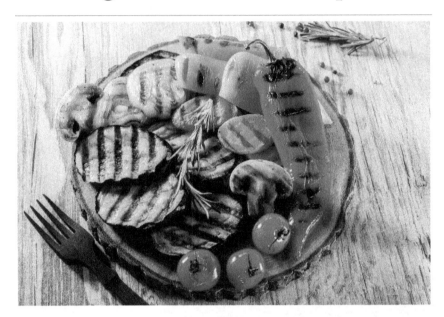

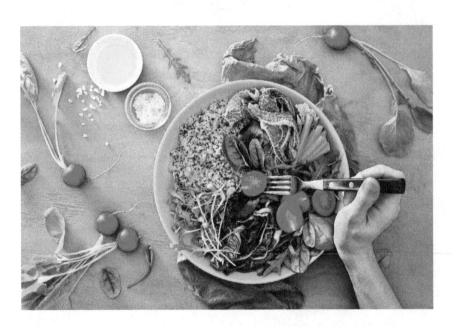

31. Kiwi Chips

Preparation Time: 5 minutes

Cooking Time: 45 minutes

Servings: 6

Ingredients:

- 1 kg kiwi
- ½ tsp. cinnamon (ground)
- ¼ tsp. nutmeg (ground)

Directions:

1. Slice the kiwi thinly. Keep them in a bowl.
2. Sprinkle nutmeg and cinnamon from the top. Toss for mixing.
3. Preheat the air fryer at 165°C.
4. Cook the kiwi in the air fryer for half an hour. Make sure you shake the basket halfway.
5. Let the chips cool down in the basket for fifteen minutes.
6. Cool before serving.

Nutrition:

- **Calories**: 110 kcal
- **Fat**: 1.1 g
- **Carbohydrates**: 26.3 g
- **Proteins**: 2.1 g

32. Apple Crisp

Preparation Time: 9 minutes

Cooking Time: 20-25 minutes

Servings: 2

Ingredients:

- 2 apples (chopped)
- 1 tsp. each
- Lemon juice
- Cinnamon
- 2 tbsp. brown sugar

For the topping:

- 3 tbsp. flour
- 2 tbsp. brown sugar
- ½ tsp. salt
- 4 tbsp. rolled oats
- 1 and a half tbsp. butter

Directions:

1. Heat your air fryer at 170°C. Use butter for greasing the basket.
2. Combine lemon juice, apples, cinnamon, and sugar together in a bowl.

3. Cook the mixture for fifteen minutes. Shake the basket and cook again for five minutes.
4. For the topping, mix sugar, flour, salt, butter, and oats. Use an electric mixer for mixing.
5. Scatter the topping over the cooked apples.
6. Return the basket to the air fryer. Cook again for five minutes.

Nutrition:

- **Calories**: 341 kcal
- **Proteins**: 3.9 g
- **Carbohydrates**: 60.5 g
- **Fat**: 12.3 g

33. Roasted Veggies

Preparation Time: 6 minutes

Cooking Time: 15 minutes

Servings: 4

Ingredients:

- ½ cup each
- Summer squash (diced)
- Zucchini (diced)
- Mushrooms (diced)
- Cauliflower (diced)
- Asparagus (diced)
- Sweet red pepper (diced)
- 2 tsps. vegetable oil
- ¼ tsp. salt
- ½ tsp. black pepper (ground)
- 1 tsp. seasoning

Directions:

1. Preheat air fryer at 180°C.
2. Mix all the veggies, oil, pepper, seasoning, and salt in a bowl. Toss well for coating.
3. Cook the mixture of veggies in the air fryer for ten minutes.

Nutrition:

- **Calories**: 35 kcal
- **Fat**: 2.6 g
- **Carbohydrates**: 3.3 g
- **Proteins**: 1.3 g

34. Sweet and Spicy Carrots

Preparation Time: 9 minutes

Cooking Time: 24 minutes

Servings: 2

Ingredients:

- 1 serving cooking spray
- 1 tbsp. each
- Hot honey
- Butter (melted)
- Orange zest
- Orange juice
- ½ tsp. cardamom (ground)
- ½ pound baby carrots
- 1/3 tsp. black pepper and salt

Directions:

1. Heat your air fryer at 200°C. Use a cooking spray for greasing the basket.
2. Mix honey, butter, cardamom, and orange zest in a small bowl.
3. Pour the sauce over the carrots and coat well.
4. Cook the carrots for twenty minutes. Toss in between.
5. Mix orange juice with the leftover sauce.
6. Serve the carrots with sauce from the top.

Nutrition:

- **Calories**: 128 kcal
- **Fat**: 6 g
- **Carbohydrates**: 17.2 g
- **Proteins**: 1.2 g

35. Air Fried Potatoes

Preparation Time: 7 minutes

Cooking Time: 62 minutes

Servings: 2

Ingredients:

- 2 large potatoes
- 1 tbsp. peanut oil
- ½ tsp. sea salt

Directions:

1. Heat your air fryer at 200°C.
2. Brush the potatoes with oil. Sprinkle some salt.
3. Place the potatoes in the basket of the air fryer and cook for one hour.
4. Serve hot by dividing the potatoes from the center.

Nutrition:

- **Calories**: 310 kcal
- **Fat**: 6.3 g
- **Carbohydrates**: 61.5 g
- **Proteins**: 7.2 g

36. Asparagus Avocado Soup

Preparation Time: 9 minutes

Cooking Time: 22 minutes

Servings: 4

Ingredients:

- 1 avocado, peeled, pitted, cubed
- 12 ounces asparagus
- ½-tsp. ground black pepper
- 1-tsp. garlic powder
- 1-tsp. sea salt
- 2 tbsp. olive oil, divided
- ½ lemon, juiced
- 2 cups vegetable stock

Directions:

1. Switch on the air fryer, insert fryer basket, grease it with olive oil, then shut with its lid, set the fryer at 425°F and preheat for 5 minutes.

2. Meanwhile, place asparagus in a shallow dish, drizzle with 1-tbsp. oil, sprinkle with garlic powder, salt, and black pepper, and toss until well mixed.

3. Open the fryer, add asparagus in it, close with its lid and cook for 10 minutes until nicely golden and roasted, shaking halfway through the frying.

4. When the air fryer beeps, open its lid and transfer asparagus to a food processor.

5. Add remaining ingredients into a food processor and pulse until well combined and smooth.

6. Tip the soup in a saucepan, pour in water if the soup is too thick, and heat it over medium-low heat for 5 minutes until thoroughly heated.

7. Ladle soup into bowls and serve.

Nutrition:

- **Calories**: 208 kcal
- **Fat**: 11 g
- **Carbohydrates**: 2 g
- **Proteins**: 4 g

Dessert Recipes

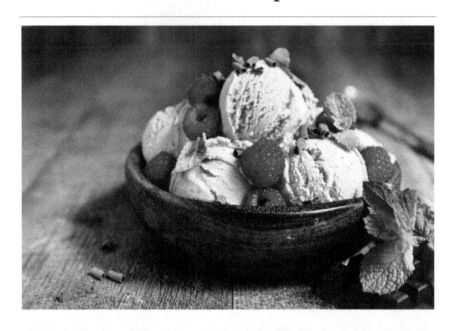

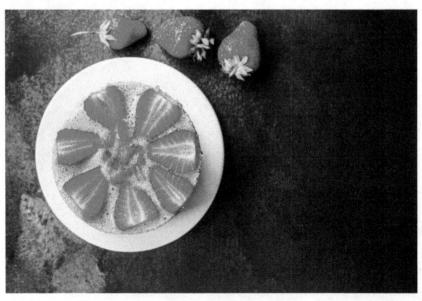

37. Sugar-Free Low Carb Peanut Butter Cookies

Preparation Time: 16 minutes

Cooking Time: 8-10 minutes

Servings: 23

Ingredients:

- 1 cup all-natural 100% peanut butter
- 1 whisked egg
- 1 tsp. liquid stevia drops
- 1 cup sugar alternative

Directions:

1. Mix all the ingredients into a dough. Make 24 balls with your hands from the combined dough.
2. On a cookie sheet or cutting board, press the dough balls with the help of a fork to form a crisscross pattern.
3. Add six cookies to the basket of the air fryer in a single layer. Make sure the cookies are separated from each other. Cook in batches
4. Let them Air Fry, for 8–10 minutes, at 325°F. Take the basket out from the air fryer.
5. Let the cookies cool for one minute, then with care, take the cookies out.
6. Keep baking the rest of the peanut butter cookies in batches.
7. Let them cool completely and serve.

Nutrition:

- **Calories**: 198 kcal
- **Carbohydrates**: 7 g
- **Proteins**: 9 g
- **Fat**: 17 g

38. Air Fryer Blueberry Muffins

Preparation Time: 9 minutes

Cooking Time: 16 minutes

Servings: 8

Ingredients:

- ½ cup sugar alternative
- 1 and 1/3 cup flour
- 1/3 cup oil
- 2 tsp. of baking powder
- ¼ tsp. salt
- 1 egg
- ½ cup milk
- 8 muffin cups (foil) with paper liners
- Or silicone baking cups
- 2/3 cup frozen and thawed blueberries or fresh

Directions:

1. Let the air fryer preheat to 330°F.
2. In a large bowl, sift together baking powder, salt, sugar, and flour. Mix well
3. In another bowl, add milk, oil, and egg mix it well.
4. To the dry ingredients to the egg mix, mix until combined but do not over mix

5. Add the blueberries carefully. Pour the mixture into muffin paper cups or muffin baking tray

6. Put four muffin cups in the air fryer basket or add more if your basket's size is big.

7. Cook for 12–14 minutes, at 330°F, or until when touch lightly the tops, it should spring back.

8. Cook the remaining muffins accordingly.

9. Take out from the air fryer and let them cool before serving.

Nutrition:

- **Calories**: 213 kcal
- **Fat**: 10 g
- **Carbohydrates**: 13.2 g
- **Proteins**: 9.7 g

39. Air Fryer Sugar-Free Lemon Slice and Bake Cookies

Preparation Time: 5 minutes

Cooking Time: 8 minutes

Servings: 24

Ingredients:

- ½ tsp. salt
- ½ cup coconut flour
- ½ cup unsalted butter softened
- ½ tsp. liquid vanilla stevia
- ½ cup swerve granular sweetener
- 1 tbsp. lemon juice
- ¼ tsp. lemon extract (optional)
- 2 egg yolks

For icing

- 3 tsp. lemon juice
- 2/3 cup Swerve confectioner's sweetener

Directions:

1. In a stand mixer bowl, add baking soda, coconut flour, salt, and Swerve, mix until well combined
2. Then add the butter (softened) to the dry ingredient, mix well. Add all the remaining ingredients but do not add in the yolks

yet. Adjust the seasoning of lemon flavor and sweetness to your liking; add more if needed.

3. Add the yolk and combine well.

4. Lay a big piece of plastic wrap on a flat surface, put the batter in the center, roll around the dough and make it into a log form for almost 12 inches. Keep this log in the fridge for 2–3 hours or overnight, if possible.

5. Let the oven preheat to 325°F. generously spray the air fryer basket, take the log out from plastic wrap, only unwrap how much you want to use it, and keep the rest in the fridge.

6. Cut in ¼-inch cookies, place as many cookies in the air fryer basket in one single, do not overcrowd the basket.

7. Bake for 3-five minutes, or until the cookies' edges become brown. Let it cool in the basket for two minutes, then take it out from the basket. And let them cool on a wire rack.

8. Once all cookies are baked, pour the icing over. Serve and enjoy.

Nutrition:

- **Calories**: 66 kcal
- **Fat**: 6 g
- **Carbohydrates**: 2 g
- **Proteins**: 1 g

40. Easy Air Fryer Brownies

Preparation Time: 9 minutes

Cooking Time: 10 minutes

Servings: 2

Ingredients:

- 2 tbsp. baking chips
- 1/3 cup almond flour
- 1 egg
- ½ tsp. baking powder
- 3 tbsp. powdered sweetener (sugar alternative)
- 2 tbsp. cocoa powder (Unsweetened)
- 2 tbsp. chopped Pecans
- 4 tbsp. melted butter

Directions:

1. Let the air fryer preheat to 350°F
2. In a large bowl, add cocoa powder, almond flour, Swerve sugar substitute, and baking powder, and give it a good mix.
3. Add melted butter and crack in the egg in the dry ingredients.
4. Mix well until combined and smooth.
5. Fold in the chopped pecans and baking chips.
6. Take two ramekins to grease them well with softened butter. Add the batter to them.

7. Bake for ten minutes. Make sure to place them as far from the heat source from the top in the air fryer.

8. Take the brownies out from the air fryer and let them cool for five minutes.

9. Serve with your favorite toppings and enjoy.

Nutrition:

- **Calories**: 201 kcal
- **Fat**: 10.2 g
- **Carbohydrates**: 14.1 g
- **Proteins**: 8.7 g

Conclusion

Using an Air Fryer can be hard at first. If you follow our tips and tricks in this book, you will cook like a pro in no time! We have listed all sorts of recipes in this book so that you can ensure that you never run out of gas while trying to make your favorite foods again! Make sure you read through the whole

This cookbook's contents were intended help you learn exactly how to do this by following step-by-step instructions that will be written for you without confusing words or often-used terms. We showed you how to prepare and cook delicious and nutritious dishes quickly and easily using an Air Fryer. You can make breakfast, lunch, dinner, snacks, and desserts using this method. You can now prepare them in under 30 minutes without storing or freezing the ingredients because the foods are not fried at all.

It is just one of the key things that you could get from this book. Along with the "how-to" instructions, you also received helpful tips and tricks to help you when cooking with an Air Fryer.

CPSIA information can be obtained
at www.ICGtesting.com
Printed in the USA
BVHW091948180521
607636BV00010B/1358

9 781801 760928